Enjoy Life While Losing Weight:
Eat what you want, believe in your body, and lose weight freely.

Jennifer P. Haely

Table of Contents

Chapter 1

Why You're Overweight: Unveiling the Complex Factors Behind Weight Gain

The struggle with excess weight is a common concern for many individuals, often leading to frustration and a search for answers. While the reasons behind being overweight can vary significantly from person to person, it's crucial to understand that weight gain is a complex interplay of various factors. In this article, we will explore some of the key reasons why you might be overweight, shedding light on both biological and lifestyle contributors.

1. Genetics and Biology
Genetics play a significant role in determining an individual's susceptibility to weight gain. Some people may have a genetic predisposition that makes it easier for them to gain weight or face challenges in losing it. Genetic factors can influence metabolism, appetite regulation, and

the way the body stores fat. While genetics can set the stage, lifestyle choices still play a crucial role in weight management.

2. Dietary Habits
The modern lifestyle has brought about a shift in dietary patterns, often leading to overconsumption of calorie-dense and nutrient-poor foods. Processed foods, high in sugar, unhealthy fats, and additives, contribute to weight gain by providing excess calories without satisfying nutritional needs. Emotional eating, consuming large portions, and mindless snacking can also lead to weight gain over time.

3. Physical Activity
Sedentary behavior is a hallmark of modern life, with many jobs requiring long hours of sitting and minimal physical activity. A lack of regular exercise contributes to weight gain by slowing down metabolism and reducing calorie expenditure. Engaging in regular physical activity not only burns calories but also improves overall health and supports weight management.

4. Stress and Emotional Factors
Stress, anxiety, and emotional factors can trigger overeating as a way to cope with negative emotions. This emotional eating can lead to weight gain over time. Finding healthier ways to manage stress, such as practicing mindfulness, engaging in hobbies, or seeking support from friends and professionals, can help mitigate this aspect of weight gain.

5. Sleep Deprivation
Poor sleep quality and insufficient sleep can disrupt hormonal balance and affect appetite regulation. Sleep deprivation can lead to increased hunger and cravings, making it challenging to maintain a healthy weight. Prioritizing regular, quality sleep can have positive effects on weight management and overall well-being.

6. Medical Conditions
Certain medical conditions, such as polycystic ovary syndrome (PCOS), thyroid disorders, and insulin resistance, can contribute to weight gain or make weight loss more challenging. It's

important to consult a healthcare professional if you suspect an underlying medical condition might be affecting your weight.

Understanding the various factors that contribute to weight gain is the first step towards making positive changes in your life. Genetics, dietary habits, physical activity, emotional well-being, sleep, and medical conditions all play a role in your weight. Recognizing that weight management is a holistic endeavor involving both biology and lifestyle choices empowers you to take control of your health. By making informed decisions and adopting sustainable habits, you can embark on a journey towards a healthier weight and a better quality of life. Remember, every individual's situation is unique, so seeking guidance from healthcare professionals or registered dietitians can provide personalized support on your weight management journey.

Coach Assignment

This week, I'd like you to take some time to reflect on the topic: "Why You're Overweight."

Remember, the goal of this exercise is not to place blame or guilt, but rather to gain insight and understanding that will help you make positive changes moving forward.

Assignment:
1. Journal Reflection: Take out your journal and find a quiet space where you can reflect. Begin by writing down your thoughts and feelings about your weight. What emotions come up when you think about it? Have you tried to lose weight before? What were the reasons behind those attempts? Be honest and open with yourself.

2. Exploring Habits: Consider the lifestyle habits that might have contributed to your current weight. Think about your eating patterns, physical activity level, sleep routine, and stress management. Are there any habits that you suspect might have led to weight gain? Write them down without judgment.

3. Emotional Connections: Often, there's an emotional component to our relationship with food and weight. Reflect on whether certain

emotions trigger overeating or unhealthy eating habits. Have there been moments when you turned to food for comfort, distraction, or celebration? Write down any emotions that you associate with your eating habits.

4. External Factors: Sometimes, external factors like work, family, or environment can play a role in weight gain. Reflect on whether any external factors have affected your ability to maintain a healthy lifestyle. Are there challenges that you've faced that might have contributed to your current weight? Write down any external factors that come to mind.

5. Positive Qualities: Shift your focus to your positive qualities and strengths. Write down qualities about yourself that have nothing to do with your weight. This can help you cultivate self-compassion and recognize that your worth goes beyond your appearance.

6. Setting Intentions: Based on your reflections, set an intention for yourself. What is one positive change you can make to move towards a healthier lifestyle? It could be related to

eating habits, physical activity, stress management, or self-care. Make sure it's a realistic and achievable goal.

Remember, this exercise is about gaining self-awareness and understanding, not about self-criticism. As you complete this reflection, keep in mind the central theme of ""Enjoy Life While Losing Weight"." Embrace the idea of trusting your body and making choices that align with your well-being.

Chapter 2

Understanding What Doesn't Work for Weight Loss: Unveiling Myths and Misconceptions

In the quest for achieving a healthy weight, there's a plethora of information available that promises quick fixes and miraculous results. However, it's essential to sift through the noise and understand what truly doesn't work for weight loss. In this article, we'll delve into common misconceptions, fad diets, and unsustainable practices that can hinder your progress on the journey towards a healthier you.

1. Extreme Diets and Fad Diets
Fad diets come and go, but they often have one thing in common: they promise rapid weight loss through extreme restrictions. Whether it's the "cabbage soup diet," "juice cleanse," or any other diet that severely limits certain food

groups, these approaches rarely lead to sustainable results. Not only do they often lack essential nutrients, but they're also difficult to maintain over the long term, leading to a cycle of weight loss and regain.

2. Skipping Meals or Severely Restricting Calories

Skipping meals or drastically cutting calories might seem like a straightforward way to shed pounds. However, this approach can backfire. Severely restricting your calorie intake can slow down your metabolism, leaving you feeling sluggish and fatigued. Additionally, skipping meals can lead to overeating later in the day due to increased hunger, which defeats the purpose of the calorie reduction.

3. Relying Solely on Supplements and Pills

The supplement industry is flooded with products claiming to accelerate weight loss without the need for dietary changes or exercise. While some supplements may have minor effects on metabolism, they can't replace a healthy diet and regular physical activity.

Relying solely on supplements often overlooks the importance of sustainable lifestyle changes.

4. Eliminating Entire Food Groups

Cutting out entire food groups, such as carbohydrates or fats, may lead to initial weight loss, but it's not a sustainable approach. Our bodies require a balanced intake of various nutrients for optimal functioning. Restricting certain food groups can lead to nutrient deficiencies and imbalances, which can harm your overall health in the long run.

5. Over Reliance on Exercise Alone

While exercise is a crucial component of a healthy lifestyle, relying solely on exercise for weight loss can yield disappointing results. Overestimating the number of calories burned through exercise and compensating with higher food intake can hinder weight loss efforts. A balanced approach that combines a healthy diet with regular physical activity is more effective.

When it comes to weight loss, it's important to separate fact from fiction and avoid falling for quick fixes that promise unrealistic results.

What doesn't work for weight loss often includes extreme diets, fad diets, skipping meals, relying solely on supplements, eliminating entire food groups, and overemphasizing exercise without dietary changes. The key to successful and sustainable weight management lies in adopting a balanced approach that focuses on nourishing your body, staying active, and making gradual, positive changes to your lifestyle.

Remember, achieving a healthy weight is a journey, and it's essential to prioritize your overall well-being rather than chasing after short-term solutions. Embrace the concepts of "Enjoy Life While Losing Weight" by nurturing a positive relationship with your body and making choices that contribute to your long-term health and happiness.

Coach Homework: Exploring What Doesn't Work for Weight Loss

" This exercise will help you identify strategies or approaches that may not have been effective in the past, so you can make more informed decisions moving forward.

Assignment:
1. Reflect on Past Attempts: Take some time to think about previous attempts you've made to lose weight. Were there any specific diets, routines, or strategies you tried that didn't yield the desired results? Write down these experiences without judgment.

2. Identify Unrealistic Expectations: Reflect on whether you've set unrealistic expectations for yourself in the past. Were you hoping for rapid results or trying to achieve an unsustainable level of restriction? Write down any unrealistic expectations you've had.

3. Examine Fad Diets: Explore any fad diets you've tried or considered. Research these diets and evaluate their promises, potential risks, and whether they align with a balanced and sustainable approach to weight management.

4. Mindless Restriction: Consider times when you've engaged in extreme calorie restriction or

eliminated entire food groups from your diet. Reflect on the impact these restrictions had on your physical and emotional well-being.

5. Neglecting Nutritional Needs: Reflect on instances where you prioritized weight loss over proper nutrition. Have you skipped meals or ignored your body's hunger signals? Write down times when you may have neglected your body's nutritional needs.

6. Overreliance on Supplements: Reflect on any instances where you relied heavily on weight loss supplements or products. Consider whether these supplements were effective in the long term or if they led to disappointment.

7. Lack of Sustainable Changes: Think about times when you made temporary changes that didn't stick. Have you tried to make drastic changes overnight that weren't sustainable in the long run? Write down these instances.

8. Ignoring Physical Activity: Reflect on whether you've neglected the importance of physical activity in your weight loss journey.

Have you underestimated the role of regular exercise in achieving and maintaining a healthy weight?

9. Emotional Triggers: Consider whether emotional triggers have led to behaviors that hindered your weight loss progress. Reflect on whether stress, boredom, or other emotions have influenced unhealthy eating patterns.

10. Positive Learnings: After reflecting on what hasn't worked, identify any lessons you've gained from these experiences. What insights can you take away to inform your approach moving forward?

Remember, this exercise is not meant to discourage you, but to empower you with knowledge. Embrace the idea that your weight loss journey is a learning process, and each experience can provide valuable insights.

Chapter 3

What Works for Weight Loss: Strategies for Successful and Sustainable Results

Weight loss is a journey that requires careful planning, dedication, and a combination of effective strategies. While there is no one-size-fits-all approach, certain methods have been proven to work for many individuals seeking to shed excess pounds. In this article, we will explore key strategies that contribute to successful and sustainable weight loss.

1. Balanced Diet:
A balanced and nutrient-dense diet forms the foundation of any effective weight loss plan. Focus on consuming a variety of whole foods, including lean proteins, complex carbohydrates, healthy fats, and a plethora of fruits and vegetables. Portion control is essential to prevent overeating while providing the body with essential nutrients.

2. Caloric Deficit:
Creating a caloric deficit, where you consume fewer calories than you expend, is fundamental to losing weight. This can be achieved through a combination of dietary adjustments and increased physical activity. Tracking your calorie intake and being mindful of portion sizes can help you maintain a consistent caloric deficit.

3. Regular Physical Activity:
Exercise plays a pivotal role in weight loss by increasing energy expenditure and enhancing overall fitness. Incorporate a mix of cardiovascular exercises (such as running, swimming, or cycling) and strength training to boost metabolism and preserve lean muscle mass. Aim for at least 150 minutes of moderate-intensity aerobic activity per week, along with muscle-strengthening activities on two or more days.

4. Mindful Eating:

Practicing mindful eating involves paying close attention to hunger cues, eating slowly, and savoring each bite. This approach helps prevent overeating, encourages better digestion, and fosters a healthier relationship with food.

5. Adequate Sleep:
Sleep is often overlooked but is crucial for weight loss success. Lack of sleep can disrupt hormones that regulate hunger and appetite, leading to increased cravings for unhealthy foods. Aim for 7-9 hours of quality sleep per night to support your weight loss efforts.

6. Hydration:
Staying well-hydrated not only aids in overall health but also supports weight loss. Drinking water before meals can help control appetite, leading to consuming fewer calories during meals.

7. Behavior Change:
Effective weight loss requires addressing underlying behaviors and habits. Identify triggers that lead to overeating or unhealthy food choices, and work on replacing them with

positive behaviors. This might involve stress management techniques, keeping a food journal, or seeking support from a counselor or support group.

8. Patience and Consistency:
Weight loss is a gradual process that requires patience and consistency. Avoid extreme diets or rapid weight loss methods, as they are often unsustainable and can lead to health complications. Aim for a gradual and steady weight loss of about 1-2 pounds per week.

The journey to successful and sustainable weight loss involves a combination of strategies, including a balanced diet, regular physical activity, mindfulness, adequate sleep, and behavior change. While there is no magic solution, embracing these principles can lead to positive and lasting results. Remember that individual needs vary, so it's essential to consult with a healthcare professional before making any significant changes to your diet or exercise routine. With dedication and a holistic approach, you can achieve your weight loss goals and enjoy improved overall well-being.

Coach Homework: What Works for Weight Loss

Assignment Overview:
In this assignment, you will explore the various factors that contribute to effective weight loss. You will research and compile a list of strategies, behaviors, and principles that have been proven to work for successful weight loss. Additionally, you will reflect on how these factors can be integrated into your own lifestyle to achieve your weight loss goals.

Assignment Tasks:

1. Research and List: Research reputable sources such as scientific studies, medical journals, and expert opinions on effective weight loss strategies. Compile a list of key factors that have consistently shown to work for weight loss.

2. Behavioral Changes: Identify specific behavioral changes that contribute to weight

loss success. These could include modifications in eating habits, physical activity, sleep patterns, and stress management.

3. Dietary Approaches: Explore different dietary approaches that aid in weight loss. Discuss the benefits of balanced and nutrient-dense meals, portion control, mindful eating, and the potential impact of fad diets.

4. Physical Activity: Examine the role of regular physical activity in weight loss. Highlight the benefits of both cardiovascular exercises and strength training, and explain how incorporating movement into daily routines can enhance weight loss efforts.

5. Lifestyle Factors: Consider the impact of lifestyle factors such as sleep, stress, and hydration on weight loss. Discuss how adequate sleep, stress reduction techniques, and proper hydration contribute to a healthier body weight.

6. Accountability and Support: Investigate the importance of accountability and social support in weight loss journeys. Explain how sharing

your goals with others, seeking professional guidance, or joining a support group can boost motivation and success.

7. Sustainable Practices: Emphasize the significance of adopting sustainable practices for long-term weight management. Discuss the drawbacks of extreme diets and the importance of making gradual, realistic changes.

8. Self-Reflection: Reflect on your own current habits and lifestyle. Identify areas where you could implement the strategies you've researched to facilitate your own weight loss journey.

Remember that the goal of this assignment is to equip you with knowledge and strategies that can contribute to your weight loss journey. Good luck!

Chapter 4

Creating a Food Lifestyle That Allows Weight Loss

Maintaining a healthy weight is not just about following a short-lived diet; it's about adopting a sustainable food lifestyle that supports your weight loss goals while promoting overall well-being. By making mindful and balanced food choices, you can create a food lifestyle that sets the foundation for successful weight loss. Let's explore key principles and strategies to help you achieve this goal.

1. Embrace Balanced Nutrition:
A successful weight loss food lifestyle centers around consuming a balanced mix of macronutrients: carbohydrates, proteins, and fats. Prioritize whole grains, lean proteins, healthy fats, and a variety of fruits and vegetables. This balance helps regulate your

metabolism and energy levels, while providing essential nutrients for your body's functions.

2. Practice Portion Control:
Portion control is crucial for managing calorie intake. Invest in smaller plates and bowls, and be mindful of serving sizes. This practice encourages you to enjoy your favorite foods without overindulging.

3. Mindful Eating:
Eating mindfully involves savoring every bite and paying attention to hunger and fullness cues. Slow down during meals, chew thoroughly, and put away distractions like screens. This practice helps prevent overeating by allowing your body to recognize when it's satisfied.

4. Hydration Matters:
Water plays a significant role in weight loss. Staying adequately hydrated can help control appetite, boost metabolism, and promote overall well-being. Aim for at least 8 glasses of water a day and consider incorporating herbal teas or infused water for variety.

5. Plan and Prep Meals:
Planning and preparing meals in advance can help you make healthier choices and avoid impulsive, less nutritious options. Batch cooking, creating a weekly meal plan, and having nutritious snacks on hand can contribute to a successful weight loss journey.

6. Be Wary of Processed Foods:
Processed foods are often high in added sugars, unhealthy fats, and artificial additives. Minimize their consumption and prioritize whole, unprocessed foods for optimal nutrition and weight loss.

7. Choose Nutrient-Dense Snacks:
Snacking can be part of a healthy food lifestyle, provided you choose nutrient-dense options. Opt for snacks rich in protein, fiber, and healthy fats, such as Greek yogurt with berries, mixed nuts, or sliced vegetables with hummus.

8. Practice Moderation, Not Deprivation:

Depriving yourself of your favorite foods can lead to cravings and setbacks. Instead, practice moderation by enjoying occasional treats without guilt. The key is to savor these treats mindfully and return to your healthier choices afterward.

9. Listen to Your Body:
Your body is unique, and its nutritional needs may vary. Pay attention to how certain foods make you feel and adjust your choices accordingly. This self-awareness helps you create a food lifestyle tailored to your individual requirements.

10. Seek Professional Guidance:
Consulting a registered dietitian or a nutritionist can provide personalized guidance and support. They can help you design a food lifestyle that aligns with your weight loss goals, taking into consideration your preferences, health conditions, and lifestyle.

Remember, creating a food lifestyle that supports weight loss is a gradual process that involves making sustainable changes over time.

By embracing balanced nutrition, portion control, mindful eating, and other key strategies, you can develop habits that not only help you shed excess weight but also promote your overall health and well-being.

Coach Homework: Creating a Food Lifestyle for Weight Loss

Assignment Overview:
In this assignment, you will delve into the development of a food lifestyle that promotes effective weight loss. You will explore various aspects of nutrition, dietary choices, meal planning, and mindful eating. Your goal is to create a sustainable approach to food that aligns with your weight loss objectives.

Assignment Tasks:

1. Understanding Nutritional Basics: Research the fundamental principles of nutrition, including macronutrients (carbohydrates, proteins, fats) and micronutrients (vitamins, minerals). Explain their roles in the body and their importance in a weight loss journey.

2. Caloric Intake and Portion Control: Investigate the relationship between caloric intake and weight loss. Discuss the significance of portion control, mindful eating, and the concept of "calories in vs. calories out."

3. Balanced and Nutrient-Dense Meals: Emphasize the benefits of incorporating a variety of whole foods into your diet. Create a list of nutrient-dense foods that can support your weight loss goals and explain how to create balanced meals.

4. Meal Planning and Preparation: Describe the advantages of meal planning in a weight loss journey. Provide tips for effective meal prep, including batch cooking, portioning, and storing meals for convenience.

5. Mindful Eating Practices: Explore the concept of mindful eating and its role in weight loss. Explain how paying attention to hunger cues, eating slowly, and savoring flavors can

contribute to better portion control and satisfaction.

6. Hydration: Discuss the importance of staying hydrated for weight loss. Explain how drinking water can support metabolism, control appetite, and aid in overall well-being.

7. Limiting Processed Foods and Sugar: Examine the impact of processed foods and added sugars on weight loss efforts. Provide strategies for reducing consumption of these items and offer healthier alternatives.

8. Eating Out and Social Situations: Address challenges related to eating out and social gatherings. Offer tips for making healthier choices in restaurants and navigating situations where unhealthy food options may be prevalent.

9. Progress Tracking and Adjustments: Explain the value of tracking your food intake and progress. Discuss how to evaluate your approach over time and make necessary adjustments for continued success.

Remember, creating a sustainable food lifestyle is key to achieving your weight loss goals. Approach this assignment as a roadmap to healthier eating habits. Good luck!

Chapter 5

Making Peace with Hunger: A Path to Mindful Eating and Well-being

Hunger is a natural and essential bodily signal that often carries deeper meanings beyond its physical implications. In a society that promotes overconsumption and instant gratification, learning to make peace with hunger is a transformative journey that can lead to a healthier relationship with food, increased mindfulness, and enhanced overall well-being. This article explores the art of embracing hunger, understanding its nuances, and redefining our connection with food.

Hunger:
More Than a Physical Sensation:
Hunger extends beyond the growling stomach and gnawing emptiness. It is a complex interplay of physiological cues, emotions, and psychological factors. Distinguishing between

physical and emotional hunger is vital in creating a harmonious relationship with our body's cues.

Mindful Eating and the Hunger Scale:
Mindful eating encourages us to reconnect with our bodies and engage our senses while consuming food. The hunger scale is a valuable tool in this journey, ranging from 1 (starving) to 10 (overly full). By tuning into our hunger level before, during, and after meals, we can make informed choices that honor our body's true needs.

Embracing the Sensation of Hunger:
1. Recognize Hunger as a Signal: Instead of fearing hunger, view it as a communication from your body. Hunger signals that your body is ready to refuel, nourish, and sustain itself.

2. Eat with Intention: When hunger arises, approach your meals with intention and awareness. Choose foods that nourish your body and align with your goals.

3. Practice Mindfulness: Engage your senses during meals. Savor the flavors, textures, and aromas of your food. Mindful eating transforms meals into moments of pleasure and nourishment.

4. Acknowledge Fullness: Listen to your body's cues of fullness. Eating beyond satisfaction can lead to discomfort and disrupt the delicate balance between hunger and satiety.

Detaching from Emotional Eating:
Recognize the difference between physical and emotional hunger. Emotional eating, often triggered by stress, boredom, or other emotions, is a temporary fix that doesn't address the root cause. Engage in activities that genuinely fulfill you instead of relying on food to soothe emotions.

Breaking Free from Diet Culture:
Diet culture often perpetuates the fear of hunger and promotes strict meal plans. Shift your focus from restriction to nourishment. Prioritize whole, nutrient-dense foods that provide sustained energy and satisfaction.

Empowerment through Intuitive Eating:
Intuitive eating centers on trusting your body's wisdom to guide your food choices. By letting go of rigid rules and external cues, you can develop a healthier relationship with food and your body.

Making peace with hunger is an empowering journey that transcends mere sustenance. It's about reclaiming our innate ability to listen to our bodies, honor our needs, and nourish ourselves holistically. By embracing hunger as a vital communication and practicing mindful eating, we can foster a harmonious relationship with food that enhances our physical, emotional, and mental well-being. Letting go of fear and embracing hunger paves the way for a life filled with mindful choices, self-compassion, and lasting vitality.

Coach Homework: Making Peace with Hunger

Assignment Overview:

In this assignment, you will explore the concept of making peace with hunger as a part of your journey towards a healthier relationship with food. You will delve into the reasons behind hunger, the various types of hunger, and strategies to respond to hunger cues in a balanced and mindful manner.

Assignment Tasks:

1. Understanding Hunger: Research and explain the physiological and psychological aspects of hunger. Describe how the body signals its need for nourishment and the different factors that contribute to the sensation of hunger.

2. Types of Hunger: Discuss the difference between physical hunger and emotional hunger. Outline the characteristics of each type and provide examples of situations that might trigger emotional eating.

3. Mindful Eating: Explore the concept of mindful eating and its role in making peace with hunger. Explain how being present during

meals, savoring flavors, and paying attention to hunger and fullness cues can promote a healthier relationship with food.

4. Listening to Your Body: Explain the importance of listening to your body's signals and cues when it comes to hunger and fullness. Offer strategies for recognizing when you are genuinely hungry and when you might be eating for emotional reasons.

5. Honoring Hunger: Discuss the significance of honoring your body's hunger signals and avoiding extreme restrictions. Address the negative consequences of ignoring hunger cues and how it can impact metabolism and overall well-being.

6. Balancing Nutritional Needs: Provide guidance on how to make nutritious food choices while responding to hunger. Explain how to create balanced meals that satisfy both physical and nutritional needs.

7. Developing Resilience: Explore strategies to cope with hunger in a healthy way. Discuss the

role of patience, resilience, and distraction techniques in managing hunger between meals.

8. Self-Reflection: Reflect on your own relationship with hunger and eating habits. Identify instances where you may have struggled with recognizing and responding to hunger cues, and consider how the strategies discussed can be applied to your own experiences.

The goal of this assignment is to help you develop a healthier relationship with hunger and eating. Remember that making peace with hunger is an essential step towards intuitive eating and improved overall well-being. Good luck!

Chapter 6

Six Habits for Achieving Consistent Weight Loss

Consistent weight loss is a journey that requires commitment, discipline, and the adoption of healthy habits. Rather than relying on fad diets or quick fixes, incorporating sustainable lifestyle changes is key to achieving and maintaining a healthier weight. In this article, we'll explore six habits that can contribute to consistent and lasting weight loss.

1. Mindful Eating:
Practicing mindful eating involves paying full attention to the present moment while consuming your meals. Focus on the flavors, textures, and sensations of the food. This habit not only enhances your eating experience but also helps you recognize when you're truly hungry and when you're comfortably full, preventing overeating.

2. Regular Physical Activity:
Incorporating regular exercise into your routine is vital for weight loss. Engage in a mix of cardiovascular activities, such as walking, running, or swimming, along with strength training to build lean muscle. Consistency is key, so find activities you enjoy to make exercise a sustainable part of your lifestyle.

3. Balanced Nutrition:
Adopting a balanced approach to nutrition is crucial for weight loss. Focus on consuming a variety of nutrient-dense foods that provide essential vitamins, minerals, and macronutrients. Prioritize whole grains, lean proteins, healthy fats, and a colorful array of fruits and vegetables to fuel your body.

4. Portion Control:
Being mindful of portion sizes can prevent overeating and support weight loss. Use smaller plates, bowls, and utensils to help control portions, and pay attention to your body's hunger and fullness cues to avoid eating beyond what you need.

5. Adequate Sleep:
Getting enough quality sleep is often overlooked in weight loss efforts. Sleep plays a crucial role in regulating hormones that control hunger and appetite. Aim for 7-9 hours of sleep per night to support your weight loss goals and overall well-being.

6. Consistent Hydration:
Staying hydrated is essential for weight loss as well as overall health. Drinking water throughout the day can help control appetite, boost metabolism, and improve digestion. Aim to drink adequate water and limit sugary beverages.

Achieving consistent weight loss requires a holistic approach that encompasses various aspects of your lifestyle. By adopting habits such as mindful eating, regular physical activity, balanced nutrition, portion control, adequate sleep, and hydration, you'll create a solid foundation for sustainable weight loss. Remember that patience and consistency are key; the journey is about making gradual changes that lead to long-lasting results. Embrace these habits as part of your daily routine, and you'll be well on your way to a healthier and happier you.

Coach Homework: Six Habits for Consistent Weight Loss

Assignment Overview:
In this assignment, you will explore and develop six key habits that are crucial for consistent and sustainable weight loss. These habits will serve as a foundation for your weight loss journey and help you achieve your goals over the long term.

Assignment Tasks:

1. Setting Clear Goals: Define your weight loss goals in specific and realistic terms. Clarify the amount of weight you aim to lose, the timeframe, and the reasons behind your goals. Reflect on the importance of having clear objectives for motivation.

2. Nutrient-Dense Eating: Research and identify nutrient-dense foods that support weight loss. Create a list of whole foods rich in vitamins, minerals, and fiber. Discuss the importance of including a variety of foods from different food groups in your diet.

3. Portion Control and Mindful Eating: Explain the concept of portion control and its role in weight management. Explore mindful eating techniques, such as eating slowly, savoring flavors, and paying attention to hunger and fullness cues.

4. Regular Physical Activity: Discuss the significance of regular exercise for weight loss. Detail the benefits of cardiovascular workouts and strength training. Outline a feasible exercise routine that aligns with your fitness level and preferences.

5. Consistent Sleep Routine: Research the connection between sleep and weight loss. Explain how adequate sleep supports metabolism and overall well-being. Develop a

sleep schedule that allows you to get 7-9 hours of quality sleep each night.

6. Accountability and Tracking: Explore the importance of accountability in weight loss. Identify methods for tracking your progress, such as keeping a food journal, recording workouts, or using apps. Discuss how accountability can motivate you to stay on track.

By cultivating these six habits, you'll be on the path to consistent weight loss and improved well-being. Approach this assignment as a roadmap for making positive changes that will benefit you in the long run. Good luck!

Chapter 7

Breaking the Habit of Overeating: Strategies for a Healthier Relationship with Food

Overeating can often become a frustrating cycle, impacting not just our physical health but also our emotional well-being. Breaking free from the habit of overeating requires a combination of self-awareness, mindful practices, and a commitment to building a healthier relationship with food. In this article, we'll explore effective strategies that can help you regain control over your eating habits and foster a more balanced approach to nourishment.

1. Cultivate Mindful Eating:
Mindful eating involves paying close attention to your thoughts, feelings, and sensations while eating. Start by slowing down and savoring each bite. Engage your senses and truly experience

the taste, texture, and aroma of your food. Mindful eating helps you tune into hunger and fullness cues, preventing the mindless consumption that often leads to overeating.

2. Identify Emotional Triggers:
Many instances of overeating are driven by emotions rather than physical hunger. Recognize the emotional triggers that prompt you to eat beyond your needs. Whether it's stress, boredom, loneliness, or sadness, identifying these triggers allows you to find alternative ways to cope without turning to food.

3. Practice Portion Control:
Portion control is crucial in managing overeating. Use smaller plates and bowls, and serve yourself appropriate portions. Avoid eating straight from a bag or container, as this can make it difficult to gauge how much you've consumed. Being mindful of portion sizes helps you become more in tune with your body's signals.

4. Establish Regular Meal Times:

Skipping meals can lead to excessive hunger and overeating later on. Aim to eat regular, balanced meals throughout the day. This helps stabilize blood sugar levels and prevents the intense hunger that often drives overindulgence.

5. Keep a Food Journal:
Keeping a food journal can help you track what you eat, when you eat, and how you feel before and after eating. This practice promotes self-awareness and highlights patterns of overeating. Reviewing your journal can provide insights into your triggers and habits.

6. Find Healthy Alternatives:
When the urge to overeat strikes, have healthy alternatives readily available. Stock your kitchen with nutritious snacks like fruits, vegetables, nuts, and yogurt. Having these options on hand makes it easier to make mindful choices when cravings arise.

7. Practice Self-Compassion:
Avoid being too hard on yourself if you slip up. Overeating occasionally is normal and does not

define your progress. Instead of dwelling on mistakes, focus on the positive changes you're making and the journey toward a healthier relationship with food.

8. Seek Professional Help:
If overeating is deeply ingrained or causing significant distress, consider seeking guidance from a registered dietitian, therapist, or counselor. These professionals can provide personalized strategies and support tailored to your needs.

Breaking the habit of overeating is a journey that requires patience, commitment, and self-awareness. By incorporating mindful practices, identifying emotional triggers, and making gradual changes to your eating habits, you can regain control over your relationship with food. Remember, it's about fostering a healthier mindset and nurturing your body with the nourishment it deserves. With determination and the right strategies, you can pave the way to a more balanced and enjoyable approach to eating.

Coach Homework: Breaking the Habit of Overeating

Assignment Overview:
In this assignment, you will explore strategies to break the habit of overeating and develop a healthier relationship with food. Overcoming overeating involves understanding the underlying causes, implementing mindful eating practices, and adopting new habits that promote balanced consumption.

Assignment Tasks:

1. Self-Awareness: Reflect on your eating habits and identify situations that trigger overeating. Consider emotional triggers, external cues, and times when you tend to overindulge.

2. Mindful Eating Practices: Research and explain the concept of mindful eating. Discuss techniques such as eating slowly, savoring flavors, and paying attention to hunger and fullness cues. Describe how mindfulness can help prevent overeating.

3. Creating a Supportive Environment: Explore ways to create an environment that supports healthier eating habits. Discuss strategies such as keeping unhealthy foods out of sight, stocking your kitchen with nutritious options, and avoiding eating in front of screens.

4. Portion Control: Explain the importance of portion control in preventing overeating. Provide tips for estimating appropriate portion sizes and using visual cues to gauge portion sizes.

5. Emotional Eating: Address the connection between emotions and overeating. Discuss alternative ways to cope with emotions, such as practicing relaxation techniques, engaging in physical activity, or seeking social support.

6. Meal Planning: Outline the benefits of meal planning in preventing overeating. Provide guidance on how to plan balanced meals and snacks in advance, which can help you avoid impulsive eating.

7. Food Choice Strategies: Research foods that promote satiety and discuss how choosing nutrient-dense foods can help prevent overeating. Explore the role of protein, fiber, and healthy fats in maintaining feelings of fullness.

8. Learning from Setbacks: Discuss the inevitability of occasional overeating episodes and how to learn from them rather than feeling defeated. Emphasize the importance of self-compassion and getting back on track.

By actively engaging in these strategies, you'll be taking steps toward breaking the habit of overeating and fostering a healthier relationship with food. Remember that change takes time, and this assignment is designed to guide you in creating sustainable habits for the long term. Good luck!

Chapter 8

Selling Yourself on Weight Loss: The Path to Personal Transformation

Embarking on a weight loss journey is not just about shedding pounds; it's a transformative process that requires commitment, determination, and a belief in your own capabilities. To embark on this journey successfully, you need to sell yourself on the idea of weight loss. This means cultivating a positive mindset, setting clear intentions, and embracing the power of self-motivation. This article will guide you through the process of selling yourself on weight loss and unlocking your full potential for personal transformation.

1. Cultivate a Positive Mindset:
Before you can effectively sell yourself on weight loss, you must shift your mindset from doubt to belief. Banish negative self-talk and replace it with affirmations that reinforce your

goals. Cultivate self-compassion and recognize that this journey is about self-improvement, not self-criticism.

2. Define Your "Why":
Dig deep and uncover the reasons behind your desire for weight loss. Whether it's improving your health, boosting confidence, or increasing energy levels, having a clear and powerful "why" will drive your motivation and commitment.

3. Visualize Success:
Visualize yourself at your desired weight and health level. Imagine the benefits of your efforts – feeling more energetic, fitting into clothes you love, and experiencing a higher quality of life. Visualization can provide a tangible goal to work toward.

4. Set Realistic Goals:
Break down your weight loss journey into achievable goals. Set both short-term and long-term objectives to maintain a sense of accomplishment throughout the process.

Celebrate your successes, no matter how small they may seem.

5. Educate Yourself:
Arm yourself with knowledge about nutrition, exercise, and healthy habits. Understanding the science behind weight loss can empower you to make informed decisions and stay committed to your goals.

6. Develop a Plan:
Craft a personalized weight loss plan that aligns with your lifestyle. Incorporate balanced meals, regular exercise, and stress management techniques. Having a structured plan provides a roadmap for success.

7. Track Progress:
Document your progress through journals, photos, or apps. Seeing how far you've come can motivate you to keep going, especially during moments of doubt.

8. Stay Accountable:
Enlist the support of friends, family, or a weight loss community. Sharing your goals and

progress with others can provide encouragement, accountability, and a sense of camaraderie.

9. Celebrate Non-Scale Victories:
Recognize that success isn't solely defined by the number on the scale. Celebrate non-scale victories, such as increased energy, improved sleep, or positive changes in your mindset.

10. Practice Self-Kindness:
Be patient with yourself and acknowledge that setbacks are part of the journey. Treat yourself with kindness and use setbacks as learning opportunities rather than reasons to give up.

Selling yourself on weight loss is about recognizing your own potential and embracing the transformation that lies ahead. By cultivating a positive mindset, setting clear intentions, and nurturing self-motivation, you can embark on a journey of personal growth and lasting change. Remember, you are capable of achieving your goals, and each step forward is a testament to your resilience and determination. Embrace this journey, and let it be a reflection of your inner strength and commitment to a healthier, happier you.